Intermittent fasting

*How Intermittent Fasting Burns Fat And Improves Your
Energy Levels Much Faster and Learn the Best Detoxification
Techniques to Improve Your Health*

Marion Fields

Published by Jason Thawne Publishing House

© Marion Fields

Intermittent fasting : How Intermittent Fasting Burns Fat And Improves Your Energy Levels Much Faster and Learn the Best Detoxification Techniques to Improve Your Health

All Rights Reserved

ISBN 978-1-989749-52-4

This document is geared towards providing exact and reliable information in regards to the topic and issue covered. The publication is sold with the idea that the publisher isn't required to render accounting, officially permitted, or otherwise, qualified services. If advice is necessary, legal or even professional, a practiced individual in the profession should be ordered.

- From a Declaration of Principles which was accepted and approved equally by a Committee of the American Bar Association and a Committee of Publishers and Associations.

In no way is it legal to reproduce, duplicate, or even transmit any part of this document in either electronic means or in printed format. Recording of this publication is strictly prohibited and any storage of this document isn't allowed unless with proper written permission from the publisher. All rights reserved.

The information provided herein is stated to be truthful and consistent, in that any liability, in terms of inattention or otherwise, by any usage or abuse of any policies, processes, or directions contained within is the solitary and also utter responsibility of the recipient reader. Under no circumstances will any legal responsibility or blame be held against the publisher for any reparation, damages, or monetary loss due to the information herein, either directly or indirectly.

Respective authors own all copyrights not held by the publisher.

The information herein is offered for just informational purposes solely, and is universal as so. The presentation of the information is without contract or any type of guarantee assurance.

The trademarks that are used are without any consent, and also the publication of the trademark is without permission or backing by the trademark owner. All trademarks and brands within this book are for clarifying purposes only and are the owned by the owners themselves, not affiliated with this document.

TABLE OF CONTENTS

PART 1 1

CHAPTER 1 – ALL ABOUT THE INTERMITTENT FASTING DIET 1

CHAPTER 2 – AN OVERVIEW OF HEALTHY FOOD CHOICES . 6

CHAPTER 3 – WEEK 1 INTERMITTENT FASTING 500 CALORIE RECIPES 13

CHICKEN SOFT TACOS 16

SERVES ONE PERSON 16

SMART BARS 17

MAKES: 4 STRIPS – ONLY EAT TWO ON YOUR FASTING DAYS 19

CHAPTER 4 – WEEK 2 INTERMITTENT FASTING 500 CALORIE RECIPES 20

SHRIMP FRIED BROWN RICE 20

PROTEIN BANANA SMOOTHIE 21

CHAPTER 5 – WEEK 3 INTERMITTENT FASTING 500 CALORIE RECIPES 23

PEPPER/STEAK TACOS 23

STUFFED CHILI AND CHEESE POTATO 24

CAJUN CHICKEN AND DIRTY RICE 25

CHAPTER 6 – WEEK 4 INTERMITTENT FASTING 500 CALORIE RECIPES 26

FLANK STEAK WITH ARUGULA SALAD AND SWEET POTATO FRIES 26

CHAPTER 7 – CONCLUSION 29

PART 2 32

CHAPTER 1: THE 5:2 DIET OVERVIEW 35

CHAPTER 2: THE SHOPPING LIST 41

FOODS THAT SHOULD BE EATEN IN GENERAL 41

FOODS TO BE EATEN IN MODERATION ON FAST DAYS 48

FOODS TO BE AVOIDED UNLESS IT'S EATEN AS A REWARD MEAL 51

CHAPTER 3: 500 CALORIES MEALS 55

SALMON FILLETS WITH MINTY PESTO 56

JAPANESE-STYLE SALMON AND VEGETABLE CURRY 58

ROASTED VEGGIES AND FETA SALAD 59

MEXICAN BURRITO 61

TURKEY RISOTTO 63

SMOKED SALMON STIR-FRY 64

CHAPTER 4: 250 CALORIES MEALS 66

CHICKEN TACO BOWLS 66

LEMON CHICKEN AND RICE STIR-FRY 68

SWEET POTATO PASTA 69

PORK AND PEPPER FAJITAS 71

CHICKEN PEPERONATA 72

LAMB ROGAN JOSH CURRY	73
CHAPTER 5: 100 CALORIES MEALS AND SNACKS	76
ASIAN CHICKEN SALAD	76
MUSHROOM STROGANOFF	77
CHICKEN BURGER AND TOMATO SALSA	79
CHORIZO AND BEAN SALAD	80
CHAPTER 6: NON-FAST DAY MEALS	84
BREAKFAST	85
FRESH MEXICAN TUNA SALAD	85
BREAKFAST BURRITO	86
LUNCH	88
ASIAN SALAD WITH CRISPY CHICKEN	88
CHICKEN MILANESE WITH ARUGULA SALAD	90
DINNER	91
GRILLED PORK CHOPS WITH CILANTRO SALSA	91
FARFALLE WITH CHICKEN AND PESTO	93
CHAPTER 7: SUCCESS WITH THE 5:2 DIET	95
CHAPTER 8: FREQUENTLY ASKED QUESTIONS	99
CONCLUSION	102
ABOUT THE AUTHOR	102

Part 1

Chapter 1 – All about the Intermittent Fasting Diet

We live in a culture that is simply filled to bursting with food choices. You can't drive down a street in most towns without running across at least a few fast food restaurants. And when you factor in the availability to get food at grocery stores, convenience stores, gas stations and even online, it's easy to see why so many people have problems sticking with a healthy diet.

While it is wonderful to live in a society where food is always readily available, we can all certainly understand why it is so difficult for people to lose weight these days. If you're a stress eater, like to eat fast foods or simply someone who opts for the most convenient choices when it's time to eat, it can be very difficult to find an eating plan that allows you to maintain control with so much food being easily obtainable.

However, if you're looking to lose weight fast, and want to do so without resorting to yet another fad diet that's almost sure to fail you over the long run, the Intermittent Fasting Diet may be just what you've been looking for. This diet plan, which is all about eating a well-balanced diet on most days, while tightly limiting calories during certain, pre-planned periods of time, has proven successful for millions of people who are serious about losing weight and getting into top shape.

From bodybuilders to professional athletes, there are lots of people who have found that intermittent fasting weight loss really is not only possible, but very easy and enjoyable. It may sound counterintuitive to think that a short period of very low calories could be easy to stick with for weight loss, but this method is remarkably powerful and very easy too.

So what is the intermittent fasting diet?

Perhaps it's best to lay out a typical intermittent fasting schedule to help you understand. Here is a brief breakdown of how I advise people to approach intermittent fasting:

- Days 1 – 5 are days where you eat slightly below your caloric maintenance. For most people this means eating between 1500 and 2000 calories.
- Day 6 is a day when you can eat a bit more than you did during the first five days. I recommend that you eat between 500 and 1000 calories more than you did during days 1 through 5.
- Day 7 is your fasting day. This is a day where you won't go completely without food, but you will limit your caloric intake to about 500 calories.

Once you get done with day 7, you start the cycle over again. The trick is in getting through that day of fasting without cheating on your diet or throwing in the towel entirely. To do this successfully, you need to have some fast recipes that you can go to when you are eating a very limited (in these case 500 calories) caloric intake.

That's where this eBook comes into the equation. Now that you understand the basics of how an intermittent fasting diet works, this eBook gives you the missing piece of the puzzle – tasty, nutritious and simple recipes that you can use on your fasting days.

The recipes that we will talk about a bit later are all 500 calorie recipes that are simple to prepare, filling and they all taste good enough to help you stick with your day of fasting for long-term weight loss success.

We'll actually discuss four full weeks of recipes that you can use as you work your way through your first month of 500 calorie intermittent fasting. Before we get to that full months' worth of low calorie recipes, though, we are going to discuss some smart food choices that you need to make while you are working through the Intermittent Fasting Diet.

It is possible to do this kind of diet using virtually any type of food. But if you really want to be as healthy, lean and fit as possible, it's best to carefully consider the foods that you eat; especially on your very low calorie fasting days. You want to get as much nutritional power as you can when you are eating just 500 calories on your fasting days.

In the next chapter we'll discuss some of the things you need to consider when you are on this diet and the power of certain food choices in regard to losing weight quickly while staying as healthy as you possibly can.

Chapter 2 – An Overview of Healthy Food Choices

As I mentioned in the previous chapter, you can choose to eat just about anything – as long as the total calories consumed only amounts to about 500 calories – on your fasting days. However, with all of that being said, it is in your best interest to make smart food choices – especially on the days where you are severely limiting your caloric intake.

You know the old saying that says, "You are what you eat!" right? Well it's true. You really are what you eat, and choosing the right foods goes a long way in maintaining health, vitality and well-being. And you can also up your chances of losing weight quickly by ensuring that the foods you eat are healthy, wholesome and nutritious.

I recommend eating a diet that is virtually free of processed foods. Try to eat foods that are whole foods. What does this mean? Well, try looking at the ingredient labels on the foods that you eat. The foods that contain one or possibly two ingredients are more than likely whole foods. But the foods that contain a huge list of ingredients have probably been processed eight ways since Sunday.

Processed foods are typically filled with sodium, high fructose corn syrup, white, refined flour and a whole host of artificial flavors, colors and ingredients that are just plain bad for your health.

I know that it's unrealistic to expect you to never eat processed foods, but you should do what you can to reduce your processed foods intake as much as possible. If you focus on eating lean protein sources, fruits, vegetables, nuts and seeds, you'll find that it's easy to avoid processed junk foods while still eating plenty of food that tastes good, fills you up and actually promotes a healthier lifestyle.

Foods to Avoid

Here are some foods that I think you should avoid like the plague while on the Intermittent Fasting Diet. Heck, I even advise that you avoid these foods for the most part even if you choose to go off the IF Diet. The more you can reduce your daily intake of these types of foods, the better you'll feel the more weight you'll lose and the better your overall quality of life will be.

Here are the foods you must avoid while you are on the Intermittent Fasting Diet:

▸ Foods with high sodium content.
▸ White flour products — white bread, pasta, etc...
▸ Fast foods — Burgers, Pizza, Tacos, etc...
▸ Foods with high fructose corn syrup.
▸ Deep fried foods.

I know that you'll want to indulge and eat some of these foods from time-to-time, and you should. Not that it's all that healthy to eat these kinds of foods, but having a sinful snack from time-to-time (preferably on your Day 6 of higher calorie eating) can go a long way in helping you to cope with the limitations you set on yourself during other days of Intermittent Fasting Dieting. Just don't overindulge on those higher caloric intake days and do what you can to avoid these foods on the other six days of your diet – especially on your day of 500 calorie pseudo-fasting.

Now that we've talked about some foods that should be avoided/consumed sparingly, let's talk about the types of foods that should make up the bulk of your diet. It's not a good idea to take a "calorie-only" approach to dieting. While it is important to monitor your overall caloric intake, it's best done in tandem with smart, healthy food choices. With this in mind, here are some of the foods that should make up the majority of the calories that you consume on a regular basis, especially on your fasting days:

- Lean beef
- Boneless/skinless chicken breast
- Eggs
- Beans
- Nuts – all varieties & raw when possible
- Fruits – all kinds, but fresh, whole and unprocessed.
- Vegetables – same as with the fruits.

You can eat some whole grains and dairy products, but do so sparingly. For example a cup of Greek yogurt every few days isn't a bad idea, but drinking a cup or two of milk or eating cheese every day is definitely not a good idea.

Always focus on eating lean proteins in combination with whole fruits and veggies. Add in some healthy, raw nuts and seeds and you'll have the foundation for a very healthy diet that will give you plenty of energy while helping you to ramp up your metabolism for super-fast weight loss.

Some people find that they lose a lot of weight simply by removing the processed and fast foods from their diets. I suggest simply removing these foods a week or two prior to jumping into the full-blown Intermittent Fasting Weight Loss plan. You might be amazed at how much weight you will lose simply by eliminating those poor food choices for a few weeks.

So if I had to write you a prescription for healthy, weight loss empowering foods, I'd say that you should make your daily eating based solidly around lean protein sources, plenty of green/leafy vegetables, a few servings of fruits for your sweet tooth and some nuts and seeds to ensure that you are getting plenty of healthy Omega fatty acids every day.

By focusing on these types of foods and eliminating the overly-processed foods that are so common in most peoples' diets you will be amazed at the results that you get. And when you use this style of eating with the Intermittent Fasting style of dieting, you'll be literally astounded at the results you get.

Be ready for lots of people asking you if you have lost weight or telling you that you look better than ever, because those are just a few of the reactions that people commonly get when they stick with the Intermittent Fasting weight loss plan for just a few weeks.

Okay, we have covered a lot of ground in just a short amount of time in this chapter. Now it's time to get things going in high gear. In the next chapters you will find a handful of 500 calorie recipes that you can use during your fasting days. The first few weeks include a few "fun" foods that make it easier to stick with your fasting days. Weeks 3 & 4, however, include leaner/meaner recipes that will help you to really hone in and shed body fat fast during the last two weeks of your first month on the Intermittent Fasting Diet.

Chapter 3 – Week 1 Intermittent Fasting 500 Calorie Recipes

We are finally here! You are now going to find some quick, easy, nutritious recipes that you can use on your days of 500 calorie fasting. By design, I've included only recipes that are practical, easy to make in just a few minutes and tasty enough to satisfy your cravings on those days when you're choosing to eat a lower calorie menu.

Please keep in mind that even with the best recipes on hand for these days that very low calorie dieting/fasting requires you to be disciplined and focused. Most of us have conditioned our bodies to expect thousands of calories on any given day. As such, the body will sometimes fight you in your quest to fast and lose weight. Remind yourself of these facts, and that your fasting day is only 24 hours, before you begin.

Here are few fast tips that will help you stick with it on your fasting days too:

- Double up on your water intake. Every successful weight loss plan should involve you drinking plenty of water each day. At a minimum you should drink 12 cups of water during your days of fasting on lower calorie meals.
- Include plenty of extra green vegetables if you get too hungry. While we are making every effort to stay at the 500 calorie limit on the days when you fast, you can add a cup or two of green leafy vegetables to fill up your stomach if you get intense hunger pangs.
- Take it easy on your fasting days. Don't schedule any intense exercise sessions on the days when you limit your caloric intake. You can stay active, but don't do any running, weight lifting or strenuous physical activity.
- Fruits should be limited on fasting days. While I always encourage you to

eat lots of fresh fruits, since your fasting day is all about keeping your caloric count nice and low, eating more than a cup or two of fruit may push your caloric level up a bit too high. Use extreme moderation when adding any fruits to your fasting day eating plan.

Keep these tips in mind as you begin you fast days. This information can help to give you an edge and will undoubtedly make your fasting days a bit easier to get through. After you have a few fast days under your belt, however, you'll find that getting through these days gets easier and easier. In fact, if you're like lots of other people who stick to intermittent fasting weight loss plans, you may find that you decide to introduce an extra day of fasting into the mix now and again.

Now we are ready to get onto the good stuff – your 500 calorie recipes for the first week. I'll give you a few recipes to choose from. If you don't like one, you can always try one of the others.

Chicken Soft Tacos

Serves one person

Ingredients
3 ounce grilled skinless chicken breast
Two 6" corn tortillas
One fourth cup black beans
Shredded lettuce, tomato, onion, salsa
One fourth rice, brown or Spanish
One fourth cup avocado, cubed
Extra virgin olive oil cooking spray

Directions

Spray the chicken breasts with extra virgin olive oil and grill until done. Wrap the grilled chicken into a warmed tortilla and stuff with lettuce, onion, tomato, avocado and salsa. Eat this one with some rice and black beans on the side. To get a similar meal from restaurants order two chicken soft tacos without cheese, sour cream or any extras other than salsa. You can also substitute the chicken with shrimp, fish or lean beef.

Smart Bars

This recipe makes 32 bars. You can freeze them to eat throughout the week as a snack or eat two or three bars on your fasting days.

Ingredients
1 cup quick-cooking oats
One half cup sunflower seeds
One half cup toasted wheat germ
2 large eggs
1 ripe banana, peeled and cut into chunks
One half cup dried apricots
One half cup pecan halves
One half cup raisins
One half cup dried cranberries
One half cup instant nonfat dry milk
One fourth cup whole wheat pastry flour
1 teaspoon cinnamon

One third cup maple syrup
1 teaspoon vanilla extract

Directions

1. Preheat the oven to 350ºF. Coat a 9 × 13-inch baking pan with nonstick spray.
2. Mix the oats, sunflowers seeds, apricots, pecans, raisins, cranberries, dry milk, flour and cinnamon with your food processor until all ingredients are finely chopped. Then add the syrup, banana, eggs and vanilla and give everything one final mix.
3. Transfer the mixture to the pan, wet your fingertips with cool water, and push down to make everything level. Bake until the mixture is golden brown and firm to the touch, this takes just about 20 minutes.
4. Cool in the pan and cut into 32 bars.

Honey-Mustard Turkey Strips

Makes: 4 strips – only eat two on your fasting days

Ingredients
One fourth cup Dijon or yellow mustard
2 tablespoons honey3/4 cup plain whole wheat dried bread crumbs
1 one half teaspoons reduced-sodium soy sauce
1 pound boneless skinless turkey breast, cut into strips

Directions
1. Preheat the oven to 400ºF. Spray a baking sheet with a healthy nonstick spray.
2. Use a whisk to combine the honey, mustard and soy sauce in a small bowl. Put the bread crumbs on a paper plate. Dip the turkey strips into the mixture and then roll in the bread crumbs. Spray the strips with the nonstick spray and bake at 400 degrees for 20 to 25 minutes.

Chapter 4 – Week 2 Intermittent Fasting 500 Calorie Recipes

Tortilla & Cheese Chili

Ingredients
1 and one half cups vegetarian chili
2 tablespoons chopped scallions
2 cups mixed greens
8 tortilla chips, broken
2 tablespoons shredded cheddar cheese
1 tablespoon low-fat Italian salad dressing

Directions

Warm up the chili and top with scallions, a bit of cheese and the broken tortilla pieces. Serve with a large green filled salad for a fun, filling lunch or dinner.

Shrimp Fried Brown Rice

Ingredients
1 cup cooked brown rice

1 garlic clove, minced
1 tablespoon sesame oil
1 tablespoon low-sodium soy sauce
1 tablespoon grated ginger
3 ounces precooked shrimp
2 cups bok choy or kale

Directions

Sauté the first five ingredients and then add the shrimp and bok choy/kale. Cook for about five minutes in your skillet on a low-to-medium heat setting.

Protein Banana Smoothie

Ingredients
1 serving vanilla whey protein
1 cup sliced banana
1 serving chocolate almond milk
1 serving flaxseed oil

Directions

Peel and chop the banana and put in the blender.
Add one scoop of vanilla whey protein mix.
Add a half cup of crushed ice.
Add a tablespoon or two of flaxseed oil
Blend it all until it is smooth and drink.

Chapter 5 – Week 3 Intermittent Fasting 500 Calorie Recipes

Pepper/Steak Tacos

Ingredients
1 tablespoon olive oil
1 teaspoon cumin
1 garlic clove, minced
3 ounces steak strips (use round steak with very little visible fat)
1 one half cups sliced green and red bell peppers
One half cup sliced onion
2 small (6-inch) whole-grain tortillas
4 tablespoons salsa
2 tablespoons low-fat sour cream

Directions

Sauté the olive oil, garlic and cumin for one minute in a skillet. Add the steak strips and cook for about 5 minutes on a low/medium heat level. Add the pepper and onions and cook for about 10 more minutes. Put it all together in a tortilla, top with salsa/sour cream and enjoy.

Stuffed Chili and Cheese Potato

Ingredients
1 medium potato
One half cup turkey or vegetarian chili
2 cups chopped broccoli
One fourth cup shredded cheddar cheese (optional)

Directions
Microwave bakes the potato for 5 to 7 minutes. Wrap the potato in foil and let it sit for 5 minutes. In a pot warm up the chili and chopped broccoli. Cut the potato lengthwise and top with the chili/broccoli mixture. Sprinkle cheese on top if you want to for a bit of additional flavor and cheesy texture.

Cajun Chicken and Dirty Rice

Ingredients
1 teaspoon dried Cajun seasoning
4 ounces chicken breast
2 teaspoons olive oil
2 garlic cloves, minced
1 cup chopped onion
1 green bell pepper, diced
2 tablespoons tomato paste
Few dashes Tabasco sauce, to taste
3/4 cup precooked brown rice

Directions
Sprinkle the seasoning on the chicken and bake or grill until done. Add oil to the skillet and sauté the onion, pepper, tomato paste, garlic and Tabasco sauce together for three minutes. Add the precooked wild rice and sauté for another 5 minutes. Serve it all on top of the chicken.

Chapter 6 – Week 4 Intermittent Fasting 500 Calorie Recipes

Apple Peanut Butter Crunch Dessert Treats Double up on the recipe for 400 calories. You can eat 2.5 of these on your fast days or mix with part of another recipe as your low calorie desert.

Ingredients
1 medium apple
One half tbsp. peanut butter
One half cup cereal – try Fiber One Original Cereal

Directions

Cut the apple into four slices and spread the peanut butter on. Coat with the cereal for a crunchy, sweet snack that takes just a few minutes to make.

Flank Steak With Arugula Salad and Sweet Potato Fries

Serves 2 at about 390 calories per serving

Ingredients
One half tbsp. olive oil
8 ounce. Flank steak
1 teaspoon. Kosher salt
One half teaspoon. Black pepper
1 5-ounce. Bag arugula

For the sweet potato fries:
1 sweet potato
2 teaspoon. Olive oil
Salt and pepper to taste
Cooking spray

Directions

1. Preheat the oven to 400 degrees F.
2. Cut the potato into one inch sticks and coat them with salt, pepper and oil. Coat the baking sheet with healthy nonstick spray and spread the potato slices in a single layer. Bake them until they are golden brown and crispy. Takes about 35 minutes.

3. While the potatoes are cooking, heat oil in a large skillet over a high heat. Season your steak with salt and pepper. Cook for 2 to 3 minutes per side.
4. Transfer to the oven and cook for about 8 minutes for medium-rare steak. You can cook longer if you like yours well done.
5. Put all the food together and drizzle

Chapter 7 – Conclusion

There are literally hundreds of recipes that you can experiment with for your fasting days. The Intermittent Fasting Diet does not require you to stick with any set list of recipes, so feel free to experiment and try new things. On some fasting days I might eat simply two chicken breasts (about 400 calories), a large green salad (practically no calories) and a tablespoon of natural almond butter (about 100 calories). Yes, that's a pretty plain, ordinary day of eating, but those kinds of simple culinary creations work in a pinch.

The main thing that you'll want to do is to keep an eye on your caloric intake. Try your best to stay at around 500 calories on the days when you are in full-on fasting mode. You can, of course, use week 4 recipes during week 1 and vice versa. Don't be afraid to mix things up and to have a bit of fun trying new foods during your fasting days.

And remember the importance of eating just a bit more than usual on the days prior to your fasting day. Day 6 is all about having a bit of fun and to fill your belly a bit more than usual before you go all out and reduce your caloric intake to 500 calories.

Stick with it and try to find some other low calorie recipes to try out on your fasting days. Drink plenty of water and use those green leafy vegetables to fill up when you're already near your caloric limit for the day but want to stave off those hunger pangs.

Try the Intermittent Diet Plan out for four weeks and I think you'll be amazed at the results. And if you do this diet plan in conjunction with exercise (like I recommend in my Intermittent Fasting Diet eBook) you'll see the body fat melting away like you never dreamed was possible.

Good luck on your journey to a slimmer, trimmer, healthier YOU!

Part 2

Introduction

According to the World Health Organization, since 1980 worldwide obesity has more than doubled and in 2014, over 1.9 billion adults were overweight. This fact has me concerned and I know I'm not the only one. Growing up in an environment and household where health wasn't a priority made me apart of that statistic. Changing my life around and making health, fitness and wellbeing major priorities opened my eyes to a better and more fulfilled life. But enough about me and let's focus on you. What is it that you want? Are you at a place in life where you're not comfortable in your own skin? I've been there and I know how it feels. If you want to change your life around and begin sculpting a body that suits you best then you're in the right place. I know you don't want to be a part of the statistics and the 5:2 diet can be your success tool.

The 5:2 diet is perfect for anyone who wants to lose weight without placing themselves under too much pressure immediately. Other diets can be very difficult to stick to and that's simply because it is hard to follow very precise instructions everyday without a break. The 5:2 diet however, makes failure almost impossible and I'm not saying that only to get your attention but mainly because it is true. This diet actually let's you be on a "diet" for 2 days within the week and the other 5 days you basically go back to your usual routine. How can you say no to something like that? Dieting shouldn't be difficult, well at least for long periods of time.

If you want to lose weight, become healthier, have that life changing success then make the life changing decision and follow the instructions within this book. Weight loss shouldn't be a problem and with the right information it won't be. Fortunately all the right information on the 5:2 diet can be found here in this book.

Chapter 1: The 5:2 Diet Overview

What is the 5:2 Diet?

Popularized by Dr. Michael Mosley in 2012 the 5:2 diet also known as the fast diet uses intermittent fasting to promote better health and weight loss. The diet involves fasting for 2 non-consecutive days in the week while the other 5 days the dieter can consumer normal meals with no restrictions. The idea of fasting may mean eating almost nothing throughout the day and that is a fearful idea to many but the 5:2 diet can be practiced and done with ease. On the 2 days of fasting during the week a total of 500 calories can be consumed by women and up to 600 calories for men. Cutting down your calorie intake to one quarter of the usual consumption may not seem very workable but with the right knowledge (which this book teaches) the process can be easily conquered.

Unlike other diets the 5:2 diet isn't at all complicated and the results that you can achieve with only 2 days of fasting per week is unheard of. Like seriously, how many other diets don't restrict you from eating your favorite meals for 5 days within the week? Although the diet is only now gaining popularity fasting in itself is not anything new. At the time of this book's publishing there has been decades of research done by scientists on the concept of fasting. The benefits of fasting are numerous based on discoveries made throughout the years and I'm sure there are still more to be discovered.

Why the 5:2 Diet Works?

People may ask isn't cutting calories so drastically dangerous? On the contrary we've been doing this for thousands of years but it's only now mainstream. Our early ancestors lived in a period where people would hunt their meal, kill and eat it, then eat close to nothing until the next hunt. But were they weak people?

Definitely not and that's because this practice actually made them stronger due to the stress/strain it placed on the body. I know you're thinking "since when is stress good," but in a situation like this it is. Religions all over the world practice fasting. Mark Twain even stated "A little starvation can really do more for the average sick man than can the best medicines and the best doctors."

The process is similar to that of exercising. When you do have an intense workout regime your body is placed under an enormous amount of stress and strain where muscles are ripped and torn but we all know that exercise no matter how intense it may be is a good thing when done right. After the workout when your body is given a chance to rest, recovery takes place and your muscles are rebuilt better and stronger. Fasting works in the same way where your body is placed under some stress but the recovery process that takes place after rebuilds your health to be better and stronger. And don't forget the weight reducing effects that occur during the couple days of fasting.

Now that I've removed any confusion around whether or not fasting is safe let's look more into how it relates with weight loss. Fewer calories consumed mean an increase in your metabolism hence an increase in burning fat reserves. Honestly I don't think there is any other diet that is simpler than the 5:2 diet and anyone can see how weight is lost with fasting. According to studies both recent and past the common weight loss on this diet is approximately a pound a week but others have experienced up to 3 pounds lost per week. Wow right? You're on a diet for only two days for a week and you're able to shed off an entire pound or more of body fat. Again wow right? And don't forget no muscle loss occurs during your fasting period.

Benefits of the 5:2 Diet

The 5:2 diet in particular has not have had the extensive research done on it as other diets have but fasting, the broaden topic has had enough research done that shows very promising results. Improved health in many areas have been seen with the studies done on the benefits of fasting, more specifically benefits including reduce risk of cancers, diabetes and heart diseases. The evidence which supports this was published back in 2007 and again in 2012 a separate study on fasting to control weight loss revealed that intermittent fasting could also reduce the risk of breast cancer. Other reasons why this diet is now gaining in popularity is due to the weight loss supporting evidence it has shown to have. Surely weight loss is always a huge benefit with most diets and the 5:2 diets is no exception. As mentioned before with only two days of fasting practitioners of the 5:2 diet have seen results up to 2 – 3 pounds of fat lost per week.

Life expectancy is also another big area that's included as a benefit of the 5:2 diet. IGF-1 is a chemical produced by the body which is said accelerates the aging process thus increasing aging related diseases such as type 2 diabetes and cancer. What does this have to do with anything?

Intermittent fasting lowers the IGF-1 chemical in the body which suggests that the effect of the chemical is reversed.

Is the 5:2 Diet for Everyone?

Although the diet is used by many there are certain groups of people who are advised to not practice this diet. Those who should not practice the 5:2 diet or fasting for that matter are as followed.

- Underweight individuals
- People with eating disorders
- Pregnant or women who are breast feeding
- Children and teenagers
- Type 1 or type 2 diabetics
- Individuals recovering from surgery

Chapter 2: The Shopping List

So far you have a good idea of what the 5:2 diet is all about but this chapter will tell you know exactly what you should eat in order to get the best results from the fast diet. Although you have 500 – 600 calories to work with on each of the two fasting days out of the week that doesn't mean that your choices of what to eat is as limited as the calories. As we develop the list of foods we should and shouldn't eat I will categorize the foods making it a lot simpler to be guided accordingly throughout your weight loss journey. Foods will be divided into 3 major categories which include foods to eat, foods to limit and foods to evade. Let's begin:

Foods to Eat

Foods that should be eaten in general

Protein- Low Sodium, High Protein Foods

High protein foods are essential to this diet as it helps manage weight loss and maintain muscle mass but what we are looking for are lean, low sodium foods that are high in protein. Being that the foods will be of low sodium it will help keep your blood pressure under control and also benefit with heart health. According to the U.S Food and Drug Administration low sodium foods are those with no more than 140 milligrams of sodium per serving. High protein foods however are foods with 10 grams of protein per serving. Foods following these criteria are meats, poultry, sea-food and soy products. Here's more:

- Beef – flank steak (lean), roast beef (low-sodium), round steak, cube steak, ground beef (95% lean), tenderloin steak, sirloin steak (extra lean),

- Game meats – venison, elk
- Pork – Tenderloin, pork loin, pork chopsPoultry – skinless chicken breast (boneless), skinless chicken thighs, ground chicken breast, duck breast, roasted turkey breast (low-sodium deli), skinless turkey breast (not deli), ground turkey (99% fat-free)
- Fish – Catfish, flounder, grouper, haddock, snapper, halibut, cod, sockeye salmon, sardines, sea bass, sole, swordfish, tilapia, tilefish, trout, yellow-fin tuna, branzino
- Shellfish - lobster, shrimp, clams
- Dairy - cottage cheese, swiss cheese, egg substitutes, egg whites, milk (2%), Greek yogurt (nonfat, plain)
- Powdered Protein - hemp protein, whey protein, soy protein, egg protein, rice protein
- Vegetable Protein - textured vegetable protein, tofu (for vegetarians, meat can be replaced with tofu in any meal)

Healthy Fats

Bad fats, good fats, healthy fats, saturated fats, unsaturated fats are all names we may have come across in other diets and it can be a little confusing at times keeping track of it all but don't worry because it will all be clear what foods contain the right fats (unsaturated fats) in this section. Here's a look:

- Dairy – cheeses – brie, cream cheese, blue cheese, egg yolk, feta cheese, mozzarella, romano, parmesan, goat cheese, cheddar, colby, gouda, havarti, muenster, swiss
- Dressings – creamy dressing, mayonnaise
- Fruit – avocado, olives
- Nuts and seeds – almonds, peanut butter, pecans, sesame seeds, sesame butter, hazelnuts, sunflower seeds, walnuts, macadamia nuts
- Oils – flaxseed oil, vegetable oil, olive oil, canola oil

- Other – sour cream, cream, salmon (omega 3), sardine (omega 3)

Vegetables

We all know how important vegetables are in any diet due to its vast range of health benefits. Vegetables are filled with vitamins, minerals, fiber and antioxidants which all help in maintaining a healthy diet. Vegetables however, are divided into two groups; non-starchy vegetables and starchy vegetables. Non- starchy vegetables are ideal for fast days because they're lower in carbs and are a good source of fiber whereas starchy vegetables are more suited for non-fast days since they contain more carbs than their counterpart.
- Non starchy vegetables – artichokes, asparagus, baby corn, beans (green, wax, Italian), broccoli, brussels sprouts, cabbage (green, bok choy, Chinese), cauliflower, celery, chicory, collard greens, cucumber, endive, eggplant, endive, escarole, fennel, garlic, kale,

kohlrabi, leeks, lettuce, mushrooms, mustard greens, okra, onions, peppers, parsley, radicchio, radishes, rhubarb, romaine, scallions/green onions, shallots, snow peas, spinach, sprouts, squash, swiss chard, tomatoes, turnips, watercress, zucchini

Flavorings/Condiments

What makes diets tasty and actually enjoyable? There might be more than one way to answer that question but flavorings are a major contributor to that answer. Flavorings and condiments add dimension to your meals but they're food too so be weary of the calories that are included. Condiments are a great way to add variation to dishes so the following list will be a guide to help you make the better choices when dealing with flavorings, sauces and condiments.

- Herbs and Spices– basil, bay leaves, cajun seasoning, chives, cilantro,

cayenne pepper, cumin, fennel seeds, garlic powder, ginger, Italian seasoning, mint leaf, paprika, parsley anise, rosemary, steak seasoning, thyme
- Butter spray, extracts (e.g. almond extract, maple extract, peppermint extract, vanilla extract), hummus, hot sauce, lemon juice, lime juice, low-sodium broth, low-sodium ketchup, mustard, salsa, sauces (e.g. chili paste, chili sauce, horseradish sauce, low sodium cocktail sauce, low-sodium soy sauce, tomato paste, tomato sauce, vinegar, steak and Worcestershire sauce)
- Salad dressings – look for low fat - balsamic vinaigrette, French dressing, Italian dressing
- Sweeteners – stevia (e.g. SweetLeaf, Truvia), sugar alcohols (xylitol, sorbitol, erythritol), raw local honey

Beverages

We all have one or two beverages that we enjoy almost on a daily basis and some are really healthy but as you know there are those that can be harmful when consumed frequently. The "right" kind of beverages can work with your body and supply a range of nutritional benefits which is just what you need to compliment the new habit you're trying to form. And apart from the nutritional value they offer they're a satisfying way to enjoy the little moments in life so here's a list that will make choosing the "right" beverages a lot easier.

- Water (sparkling or flat)
- Infused water (adding sliced or crushed fruit such as berries to a cold class of water)
- Milk – unsweetened almond milk, unsweetened soy milk, reduced fat milk
- Coffee or tea (including herbal)
- Coconut water (pure)
- Tomato juice

Foods to Limit

Foods to be eaten in moderation on fast days

Fruits

Fruits are nature's candy and can be substituted with sweets to; 1. Curb cravings and 2. Supply your body with its daily nutrients. Fruits are a great source of vitamins and minerals especially vitamin A and vitamin C which are essential to good health. I'm sure you've heard the phrase "an apple a day keeps the doctor away" and there's so much truth to that saying so why not have an apple a day or a fruit from the following list for that matter.

- Apples, apricots, avocadoes, berries (blackberries, blackcurrants, blueberries, cherries, cranberries, strawberries), cantaloupes, grapes, grapefruits, kiwifruits, kumquats, lemons, limes, mangoes, oranges, papayas, peaches, pears, pineapples, plums, tangerines, watermelon

Carbs

Carbs must be eaten in moderation and sticking to the "healthy" carbs is what's recommended. These carbs include legumes, grains and others. Use the list below to guide you.
- Breads – brown rice tortillas, corn tortillas, Ezekiel 4.9 breads, Joseph's lavash bread, Ezekiel 4.9 English muffin, Ezekiel 4.9 tortillas, whole-grain bread, Joseph pita bread
- Cereal – All-Bran, Fiber One, , Ezekiel 4.9 Sprouted Whole Grain, Kashi Go Lean, Kashi Good Friends Cereal, Kashi Heart to Heart, low-fat granola, oat meal, Purely Elizabeth ancient granola steel-cut oatmeal
- Grains – amaranth, barley, bran, buckwheat, brown rice, bulgur, couscous (whole wheat), farro, millet,

oats, popcorn, quinoa, spelt, wheat berry, whole wheat, wild rice
- Pasta – brown rice pasta, couscous, whole grain pasta, whole wheat pasta

Vegetables
- Starchy vegetables – corn, green peas, pumpkin, plantain, butternut squash, Legumes(lentils, soybeans/edamame, slightly salted soy nuts), root vegetables (beets, carrots, taro, parsnips, potatoes, rutabagas, sweet potatoes)

Foods to Avoid

Foods to be avoided unless it's eaten as a reward meal

Process or Refined Carbohydrates

Refined carbs are forms of sugars and starches that have been altered by means of processing and should be avoided for better health. Compared to complex carbs refined carbs are rapidly absorbed into the bloodstream which can result in surges in your blood sugar level and increased insulin levels. There's not much good that refined carbs provide other than temporarily pleasing your taste buds and we all have seen the effect of having either to many servings of cake, cookies or any other form refined carbs present themselves in. Fortunately these forms of carbs are easy to spot and here are a few you can start eliminating in meals for an improved health.

- Fruit juices
- Baked goods/snacks – including bagels, cake, chips, cookies, crackers, pretzels, donuts, pastries, pies
- Table sugar/white sugar
- Deserts

- Refined flour/white flour (foods made from dough such as pizza)
- White rice

Processed Foods

Processed foods may be of a larger range than you think. When you think of a processed meal a quick microwave meal may come to mind but the scope that they cover are many times larger than that. Any food that has been altered in some way from its natural state can be considered to be processed. These foods may contain extra sodium, fat and sugar that you don't know about and can really cause some serious health issues that you may not even realize until it's almost too late. One of the benefits of cooking from scratch is that you know exactly what is in your meal which is why homemade meals should override trips to local fast food restaurants.

- All forms of processed foods (if you do get processed foods make sure it is low sodium)

Foods high in Fat, Sugar and Salt

Foods containing unhealthy fats, added sugar and salt can definitely stimulate your taste buds even to the point where the brain can't register when you've had enough and an addiction begins to form. All these when taken more than that is needed can result in obesity, high blood pressure, stroke, heart attack and other harmful illnesses. Being able to combat these diseases by limiting the amount of sugar, salt and unhealthy fats that you consume are some of the best ways to increase health across the board. Here's what to avoid:

- Hydrogenated oil
- Fried foods
- Foods containing added sugar
- Foods high in sodium – less than 150mg per 100g is ideal

Alcoholic Beverages

We've all had that one friend who one time drunk too many alcoholic drinks and had to be brought home earlier than planned; God forbid you were that friend but the point is clear. Alcohol can take a serious toll on your body and mind making harming you in more ways than one. Alcohol has negative impacts on the brain, liver, heart, immune system, pancreas and many more areas making it difficult to function smoothly. With the 5:2 diet alcohol is a no-no and should be kept out of the house if you're easily tempted to have a drink or two.

- All alcoholic beverages – including strong liquor, wine, beer

Chapter 3: **500 Calories Meals**

The fast diet is one which is very flexible, and by that I mean you can change what you eat on fast days to suite your preference. Some like spreading their 500 calories into small meals eaten throughout the day while others rather eat one full 500 calorie meal for the day. The way in which you choose to consume your 500 calories on fast days is up to you and there's no right or wrong way either. In this chapter however, I will be addressing those who prefer one full meal on their fast day by listing amazing recipes that are best suited for this approach.

Salmon Fillets with Minty Pesto

Serves: 4
Calories: 489

Ingredients
- 4 – 6 ¼ oz (175g) salmon fillets
- 2 tbsp extra virgin olive oil and extra for brushing
- 1 lemon
- Large pack fresh mint (leaves removed)
- 3 ½ 0z (100g) bag rocket

- 1 ¾ oz (50g) grated Pecorino cheese
- 1 oz (30g) toasted cashew nuts

Directions

Step 1: using the extra virgin oil lightly brush both sides of the salmon fillets.

Step 2: heat a non-skillet pan and add the salmon fillets to cook for 5 minutes without moving them.

Step 3: turn the salmon fillets over to the other side and cook for another 5 minutes, Then squeeze over the fillets ½ of the lemon juice.

Step 4: in a food processor add in the mint, a handful of the rockets, the other ½ of the lemon juice and the roasted cashews to be finely chopped for the pesto. Add the 2 tbsp of extra virgin oil and 2tbsp of water to the mixture, then season and blitz to combine. Stir in the pecorino.

Step 4: Serve the salmon with the rockets and the pesto. Add the lemon wedges to the plate and enjoy!

Japanese-style Salmon and Vegetable Curry

Serves: 4
Calories: 457

Ingredients
- 4 – 4 ½ oz (125g) salmon fillets
- 2tbsp sunflower oil
- 1 sweet potato, peeled and chopped
- 2 tbsp teriyaki sauce
- 1 small cauliflower, cut into florets
- 7 oz (200g) green beans
- 250ml hot vegetable stock
- 3 ½ oz (100g) Chinese curry paste (Blue Dragon if possible)

Directions
Step 1: add 1 tbsp sunflower oil to a skillet and heat. Add the chopped potato to the skillet and let fry for 4-5 minutes.
Step 2: pour over the vegetable stock and curry sauce. Leave to simmer, covered, for 10-15 minutes until the potato is almost done cooking.

Step 3: add the cauliflower florets to the skillet and continue cooking

Step 4: grab another skillet and heat the remaining 1 tbsp of sunflower oil. Cook the salmon fillet, skin side down on a high heat for 3-4 minute or until crisp and turn the other side over to be cooked for 2-3 minutes. Spread regularly with the teriyaki sauce until the fillet is finished cooking through.

Step 5: When the salmon is almost cooked through add the beans to the curry sauce and cook until tender.

Step 6: add to a plate and serve!

Roasted Veggies and Feta Salad

Serves: 2
Calories: 473

Ingredients
- 17 ½ oz (500g) mixed root vegetables (e.g. parsnips, turnip, swede, beetroot, carrot)
- 1 tbsp olive oil

- 1 tsp za'tar or ras-el-hanout spice blend
- 1 tbsp fresh parsley (chopped)
- 1 ¾ oz (50g) bag rocket
- 4 tbsp pomegranate seeds
- 4 tbsp mixed seeds
- 3 ½ oz (100g) feta cheese (crumbled)

For the dressing:
- 1 tbsp tahini
- 4 tbsp Greek yogurt
- ½ lemon, juiced

Directions

Step 1: heat the oven to 200 *c (390 *F).

Step 2: peel the vegetables and chop them into small chunks. Add to a bowl with the spice blend and olive oil. Toss and place in the oven to roast for 20 – 30 minutes. Toss once more half way through cooking.

Step 3: add the parsley to the cooked veggies and toss until properly mixed. Separate the rocket between 2 plates and top it with the veggies.

Step 4: place all the dressing ingredients in a small bowl and mix in with water. Drizzle over the salad to your liking as well as top with the seeds and feta.

Mexican Burrito

Serves: 8
Calories: 450

Ingredients
- 1 tbsp olive oil
- 1 red onion, peeled and chopped
- 1 lb (500g) minced beef
- About 2 tbsp chopped fresh chives
- 150ml pot soured cream
- 8 flour, or corn, tortillas
- 2 tsp ground coriander
- 2 tsp ground cumin
- ½ tsp chilli flakes
- 2 tbsp sun-dried tomato paste
- 300ml (½ pint) hot beef stock
- 14 oz (400g) can pinto beans, drained and rinsed

For the guacamole:
- 2 tomatoes, chopped

- 1 red onion, peeled and chopped
- 1 avocado, stone removed, peeled and chopped
- Juice of 1 lime
- Handful of chopped fresh coriander

Directions

Step 1: in a large pan heat the tbsp of olive oil and add in the chopped onion to be cooked to soften.

Step 2: add the beef to the pan and cook for 5 minutes, stirring every now and then to brown evenly all over.

Step 3: add in the last 6 ingredients before the guacamole ingredients and simmer for 20 minutes.

Step 4: mix all the guacamole ingredients in a bowl.

Step 5: in another bowl add the sour cream and mix in the chives. Warm the tortillas while you're doing that.

Step 6: open the tortilla over a plate and top with the sour cream mix, guacamole and chilli beef. Wrap and enjoy!

Turkey Risotto

Serves: 3-4
Calories: 491

Ingredients
- 1 lb (500g) cooked turkey
- 7 oz (200g) broccoli florets (cut into small pieces)
- 3 ½ oz (100g) carrots (cut into small julienne strips)
- 3 ½ oz (100g) red pepper (cut into small julienne strips)
- 2 tbsp oil
- 1 chopped onion
- 7 oz (200g) short grain rice
- 600ml chicken stock
- 1 tsp garlic puree
- 3 ½ 0z (100g) grated cheddar cheese
- Seasoning

Directions
Step 1: for 2 minutes blanch the first 3 vegetables (broccoli, carrots, and peppers) in boiling water.

Step 2: heat the oil in a skillet and fry the onions until soft. Follow by adding the rice stir frying for 2 minutes.

Step 3: pour in the chicken stock and bring to a boil, letting it simmer for 20-25 minutes. Allow the rice to be properly cooked and the mixture to thicken forming a creamy like mixture.

Step 4: add in the tsp of garlic puree and cheese as well as the cooked turkey and seasoning and stir well combining all the ingredients.

Step 5: gently fold in the cooked veggies and enjoy!

Smoked Salmon Stir-fry

Serves: 2
Calories: 430

Ingredients
- 1 tbsp olive oil
- Thumb-sized piece of ginger (peeled and cut into fine strips)
- 1 red onion, peeled (cut into wedges and leaves pulled apart)

- 4 ½ oz (125g) tenderstem broccoli (stalks halved lengthways)
- 3 ½ 0z (100g) smoked salmon
- Freshly ground black pepper
- 1 tsp toasted sesame seeds
- Dash of soy sauce
- 4 ½ oz (125g) cooked rice noodles (for serving)

Directions

Step 1: Heat the oil in a frying pan and add in the ginger and onions. Stir-fry for 2-3 minutes.

Step 2: add the broccoli stalks to the frying pan and stir-fry for another 2-3 minutes. Follow this by adding the broccoli heads to the pan as well as 5 tbsp of hot water and let steam for a few minutes.

Step 3: tear the salmon into strips and add them to the pan to be cooked for about a minute.

Step 4: season the salmon with black pepper, soy sauce and drizzle with toasted sesame seeds.

Step 5: add the cooked noodles on a plate and top with the salmon and veggies.

Chapter 4: 250 Calories Meals

The previous chapter is directed to those who are comfortable or prefer having one decent meal a day but if you're the more-than-one-meal-a-day person then you will find this chapter more fitted for you. 250 calories isn't all that many calories for a full meal but with a few simple recipes we could make it work.

Chicken Taco Bowls

Serves: 4
Calories: 288

Ingredients
- 1 corn on the cob
- 1 tsp olive oil
- 4 corn tortillas
- 7 oz (200g) cooked chicken breast
- Coriander (handful)
- Zest and juice 1 lime, plus
- 4 jalapeños (chopped)
- ½-1 iceberg lettuce, shredded

For the dressing:
- ½-1 lime juice
- 2 tbsp light mayonnaise
- 1 tsp Heinz Sriracha Ketchup

Directions

Step 1: use a brush to coat the corn with oil and fry in a pan until tender. Then cut the kernels off of the cooked corn with a knife.

Step 2: heat the oven to 200*c (390 *F) and add in the corn tortillas. Let them stay there until just colored.

Step 3: use a jar or tumbler to shape the tortillas into a bowl. You may need to put on an oven gloves to do this. Ensure that the oven gloves are clean.

Step 4: cut the chicken into strips and place it in a bowl together with the jalapenos, coriander, zest and juice of one lime and season.

Step 5: in a separate bowl mix the dressing ingredients with a little water.

Step 6: fit the lettuce into the tortilla bowl and add in the chicken. Drizzle with the dressing and serve.

Lemon Chicken and Rice Stir-fry

Serves: 4
Calories: 205

Ingredients
- 7 oz (200g) chicken (small strips)
- 1 tbsp sunflower oil
- 7 oz (200g) cooked rice pouch
- 3 ½ Oz (100g) sugar snaps
- 3 ½ Oz (100g) frozen peas
- 3 ½ Oz (100g) sweet corn
- 1-2 spring onions (chopped)
- 1 tbsp sesame seeds

For the marinade:
- 2 tbsp tomato pasta sauce
- 2 tbsp soy sauce (reduced salt)
- 1 tsp garlic paste
- 1 tsp ginger paste
- ½ lemon juice

Directions

Step 1: add all the marinade ingredients to a bowl (non-metallic) and marinate the chicken in there until it's ready to be cooked. Ensure that you reserve the marinade for after the chicken is cooked.

Step 2: heat the sunflower oil in a deep frying pan and add the chicken to be fried. Stir-fry the strips of chicken for 3-4 minutes.

Step 3: add the sugar snaps, corn and peas to the chicken and continue stir-frying for an additional 2-3 minutes.

Step 4: throw in the rice, reserved marinade and 2 tbsp of water to the pan and stir-fry for a couple more minutes.

Step 5: drizzle over with the chopped spring onions and sesame seeds and serve!

Sweet Potato Pasta

Serves: 5
Calories: 200

Ingredients

- 10 ½ oz (300g) sweet potato (peeled and cut into small cubes)
- 10 ½ oz (300g) pasta shapes
- 3 ½ 0z (100g) frozen peas
- 2 tbsp semi-skimmed milk
- 5 ¼ oz (150g) low-fat natural yoghurt
- 1 ½ oz (40g) reduced fat Parmesan or mature cheese (finely grated)
- Ground black pepper

Directions

Step 1: heat a pot of water and add the potato chunks to the simmering water for 13-15 minutes or until tender, then drain.

Step 2: cook the pasta according to the package's directions and drain. Return the pasta back to the pan it was cooked in.

Step 3: add the frozen peas and sweet potato chunks to the pasta and stir through.

Step 4: add the milk and yogurt to the pan and stir through on a low heat for a couple minutes.

Step 5: sprinkle with cheese and ground black pepper and serve!

Pork and Pepper Fajitas

Serves: 4
Calories: 277

Ingredients
- 7 oz (200g)lean pork fillet (cut into strips)
- 1 crushed garlic clove
- 1 red and 1 green pepper (seeded and sliced)
- 1 red onion (sliced)
- 2 tbsp fajita seasoning
- Salt and freshly ground black pepper
- 2 tbsp chopped fresh chives
- Juice of 1 lime
- 8 cherry tomatoes (halved)
- 4 flat round tortilla breads
- 2 tbsp low-fat yogurt

Directions
Step 1: preheat a non-stick pan. Add the pork and crushed garlic to the pan and dry fry until sealed.

Step 2: season the pork with black pepper and salt as well as fajita seasoning.

Step 3: add the slices of green and red peppers and onion. Cook for 2-3 minutes.

Step 4: combine the chives, cherry tomatoes, and lime juice to the pan and mix well.

Step 5: spread the yogurt over the tortilla bread and add the pork and veggies over. Wrap it and serve!

Chicken Peperonata

Serves: 4
Calories: 250

Ingredients
- 2 tbsp olive oil
- 1 onion (sliced)
- 2 crushed garlic cloves
- 2 red peppers (sliced)
- 250ml chicken stock/wine
- 1 tbsp fresh oregano leaves/1 tbsp dried oregano leaves

4 ½ oz (125g) portobellini mushrooms (sliced)

Directions

Step 1: heat the oven to 190*c (370 *F). In the meantime season the chicken and cook on a large non-stick pan for 4 minutes (2 minutes each side) using 1 tbsp of olive oil.

Step 2: after the chicken has been cooked to a golden color on each side place it in a roasting tin. Put it in the oven for about 15 minutes.

Step 3: using the remaining oil fry the onion in the pan for 5 minutes to soften. Add mushroom, garlic and peppers and cook for an additional 5 minutes.

Step 4: add in the oregano. Also pour the chicken stock or wine, whichever you chose to use into the pan and bring to a boil.

Step 5: season and simmer for an extra 5 minutes.

Step 6: pour over the chicken and serve!

Lamb Rogan Josh Curry

Serves: 3
Calories: 234

Ingredients

- 7 oz (200g) lamb rump steaks (cubed)
- extra virgin olive oil
- 1 red onion (sliced)
- 1 crushed garlic clove
- 1 ¾ oz (50g) frozen peas
- 1 tbsp rogan josh curry paste
- 1 small sweet potato (cubed)
- 7 oz (200g) can tomato
- 1 tbsp tomato puree
- 200ml beef stock
- ½ red pepper (deseeded and cubed)

Directions

Step 1: spray a few times into a casserole pot with the olive oil and put to heat.

Step 2: fry the onions for about 3 minute or until soft.

Step 3: add the garlic, lamb and curry paste to the pot and cook for about 10 minute. Ensure to turn every now and then to properly brown.

Step 4: add the last 5 ingredients to the pot and cover. Let simmer for 40 minutes to get the lamb tender.

Step 5: throw in the peas and cook for an additional 3-5 minutes to warm through.
Step 6: let cool, serve and enjoy!

Chapter 5: 100 Calories Meals and Snacks

With foods around the 100 calorie mark you can experiment with a range of options and get use to the fast days even faster. Having something to munch on that's not all that much calories but still tasty is well appreciated by many and you too will like trying out fun foods to get you through fast days. I'm pretty sure you have moments when you feel for a little snack, for example maybe a muffin but one muffin alone will take up all your calorie consumption for the day but these foods won't.

Asian Chicken Salad

Serves: 2
Calories: 110

Ingredients
- 1 skinless chicken breast (boneless)
- 1 tbsp fish sauce

- 1 tbsp zest and juice ½ lime
- 3 ½ 0z (100g) bag mixed salad leaves
- Handful coriander (chopped)
- ¼ red onion (sliced)
- ¼ cucumber (halved lengthways and sliced)
- ½ chilli (deseeded and sliced)
- 1 tsp caster sugar

Directions

Step 1: place the chicken in a pot and cover with cold water. Bring the water to a boil and cook for 10 minutes.

Step 2: remove the chicken from the pan and cut it into strips. Place the chicken strips in a bowl and add the fish sauce, sugar, lime zest and juice. Mix the ingredients so that the sugar dissolves.

Step 3: in a separate container or bowl throw in the salad leaves and coriander. Top it with onions, cucumber, chilli, and the chicken breast.

Step 4: add dressing to the veggies (optional) and toss and serve!

Mushroom Stroganoff

Serves: 4
Calories: 90

Ingredients
- 1 1/3 lbs (600g) mixed mushroom
- 1 tbsp rapeseed oil
- 4 celery sticks (sliced)
- 1 large onion (sliced)
- 2 crushed garlic cloves
- 2 tsp smoked paprika
- 250ml vegetable stock
- 150ml sour cream
- Pepper

Directions
Step 1: heat the oil in a non-stick skillet adding in onion, garlic, and celery. Cook the ingredients for about 5 minute until soften.
Step 2: add the mushrooms and paprika and cook for an additional 5 minutes.
Step 3: pour the stock into the skillet and cook for another 10 minutes. At least half of the liquid should have evaporated.

Step 4: add in the sour cream and stir while seasoning with the pepper. Cook for 5 minutes over a medium heat.
Step 5: serve immediately after and enjoy!

Chicken Burger and Tomato Salsa

Serves: 4
Calories: 135

Ingredients
- 1 crushed garlic clove
- 3 spring onions (sliced)
- 1 tbsp pesto
- 2 tbsp fresh chopped mixed herbs (parsley, tarragon and thyme, etc.)
- 13 ¼ oz (375g) minced chicken
- 2 sun-dried tomatoes (chopped)
- 1 tsp olive oil

Salsa ingredients
- 9 oz (250g) cherry tomatoes (quartered)
- 1 red chilli (deseeded and chopped)
- 1 tbsp coriander (chopped)

- Grated rind and juice of 1 lime

Directions

Step 1: combine all the ingredients for the burger besides the olive oil and divide equally into 4. Flatten to form neat rounds and cover. Place in the fridge to chill for 30 minutes.

Step 2: in a non-metallic bowl combine all the salsa ingredients.

Step 3: preheat a grill. After chilling lightly brush over the burgers with olive oil and cook over the hot grill for 3-4 minutes on each side.

Step 4: serve immediately with salsa and enjoy!

Chorizo and Bean Salad

Serves: 4
Calories: 135

Ingredients
- 2 tsp olive oil
- 4 ½ oz (125g) piece chorizo ring (sliced)

- 2 shallots/1 small red onion (peeled and chopped)
- 2 sticks celery (sliced)
- 1 yellow pepper (deseeded and chopped)
- 150ml wine (white)
- 14 ½ oz (410g) can cannellini beans (rinsed and drained)
- 5 ¼ oz (150g) sun-blush tomatoes (drained)
- 4 spring onions (trimmed and sliced)
- Handful of fresh parsley/basil leaves
- Crusty bread, to serve

Directions

Step 1: heat the oil in a pan and add the sliced chorizo rings frying for about 2-3 minutes.

Step 2: add the pepper, celery, and shallots/onions and stir-fry for about 5 minutes.

Step 3: throw in the beans and stir in the mixture, then simmer for another 3 minutes to warm through.

Step 4: add the spring onion and tomato and serve in a bowl topped with fresh parsley or shredded basil leaves.
Step 5: serve with bread and enjoy!

100 calorie snacks

Fruits

- 1 cup blueberries – 83
- 1 orange – 60
- 1 cup strawberries – 46
- ¼ cup dried cranberries – 93
- 1 cup melon – 60
- 1 grapefruit – 64
- 1 small banana – 90
- 1/3 avocado – 107
- 1 cup cantaloupe – 55
- 1 medium peach – 40
- 1 medium pear – 100
- 1 cup raspberries – 60
- 1 cup blackberries – 62

Veggies

- 3 1/3 cups broccoli – 105
- 2 ½ Cucumber – 102
- 1 ¾ sweet white corn – 102
- 33 cherry tomato – 101

- 1 cup kale – 36
- 1 large carrot – 30
- 2 ½ cup cabbage – 85

Dairy

- 8 oz skim milk (o% fat) – 80
- ½ cup chocolate milk (1%) – 78
- String cheese Mozzarella – 80
- 1 non-fat Greek yogurt - 96
- ½ cup cottage cheese (1%) – 81
- 1 oz. soft goat cheese – 75
- ½ cup Blue bunny vanilla ice cream – 100
- ½ cup Breyer's no sugar added vanilla – 100

Others

- 1 cup cheerios - 100
- 1 hardboiled egg – 76
- 3 cups air popped popcorn – 99
- cheese stuffed pita pocket – 94
- 1 Nature Valley crunch bar – 59

Chapter 6: Non-Fast Day Meals

Sticking to what's required on fast days is important and although you can go back to your usual meals for the other 5 days of the week that doesn't mean you should eat any and everything. People sometimes believe that since they fasted and followed the directions on the 2 fast days in the week then its okay to eat whatever they feel like. To some extent you can but it's important to not overdo it or else you'll just put on the same weight you just lost or even worst maybe more.

The 5:2 diet teaches you to monitor what you put into your body and although emphasis is not placed on the majority of the week (the 5 non-fast days) practicing watching what you eat will benefit you further. Why stop at eating healthy and less than the usual for only 2 days when you can double or even triple your results by eating healthy throughout. That doesn't mean you can't have a slice of cake but health shouldn't be a onetime thing as many diets present it to be but a way of life, a lifestyle. To have better results go the extra mile with these delicious but healthy recipes.

Breakfast

Fresh Mexican Tuna Salad

Serves: 2
Calories: 309

Ingredients
- 1 large tuna can (400 grams/14 oz)
- 1 large chopped onion
- 1 large tomato
- 1 cup cilantro
- 1 lime

Directions

Step 1: to do before hand – place the chopped onions in a bowl and liberally add salt. Cover the onions with water and let sit for about 30 minutes. (This will remove the after taste from the onions).

Step 2: once the onions has been soaked, drain and rinse with water.

Step 3: chop the cilantro and tomatoes and combine them in a large bowl with the chopped onions.

Step 4: cut and squeeze the lime over the veggie mixture. (Use a strainer if necessary to catch any seeds for the lime).

Step 5: open the can of tuna draining the liquid and adding the tuna to the veggies.

Step 6: toss the salad ensuring the tuna is broken into bit sized pieces then serve.

Breakfast Burrito

Serves: 6
Calories: 197

Ingredients

- 1 chopped medium bell pepper (you can use half of a red and green)
- ½ Cup chopped red onions
- 3 large eggs
- 6 large egg whites (3/4 for liquid)
- 6 slices center cut low sodium bacon (chopped and cooked)
- ¾ cup reduced fat 2% sharp cheddar cheese (shredded)
- 6 whole wheat low carb tortillas
- Nonstick cooking spay

Directions

Step 1: spay the skillet with nonstick cooking spray and place on a medium-high heat.

Step 2: add the chopped peppers and onions to the pan and sauté until soft.

Step 3: reduce the heat to medium then pour in the eggs with the vegetables and stir until well scrambled and cooked.

Step 4: top the tortilla with 1/3 cup of the egg mixture followed by 2 tbsp of cheese and 1 bacon slice (chopped).

Step 5: roll it all together and enjoy with the family or wrap it up and store in the freeze for another time.

Lunch

Asian Salad with Crispy Chicken

Serves: 6
Calories: 173

Ingredients
- 2 chicken breast fillets, skinless, cut into 1" cubes
- 1 tablespoon canola oil
- 1 tablespoon sesame oil
- 3 cups shredded Savoy (curly) Cabbage, optional Napa Cabbage
- 2 cups chopped Romaine lettuce

- 1 carrot, peeled, sliced
- 2 tablespoons sesame seeds, lightly toasted

Dressing:
- 2 tablespoon honey
- 2 teaspoons Dijon mustard
- 1 tablespoon lite soy sauce, low sodium, optional Bragg's Liquid Aminos
- 1 tablespoon rice wine vinegar
- 1 tablespoon freshly squeezed lemon juice

Directions

Step 1: place a dry nonstick skillet over a medium fire and place sesame seeds in for about 5 minutes or until fragrant.

Step 2: In a medium skillet add canola and sesame oil, the chicken cubes will be cooked here on a medium-high heat for about 10 minutes or until cooked through and crispy.

Step 3: place the cooked chicken, lettuce, cabbage, and carrots in a bowl and sprinkle over with sesame seeds.

Step 4: mix all the dressing ingredients together and whisk until they all are properly combined.

Step 5: spread the dressing over the salad and mix and toss to combine.

Chicken Milanese with Arugula Salad

Serves: 4
Calories: 289

Ingredients

- 3 tablespoons olive oil (and oil for the grill)
- 4 - 6 ounce boneless, skinless chicken breasts
- ½ tbsp ground coriander
- 1 tsp kosher salt
- ½ tsp black pepper
- 3 tbsp fresh lemon juice
- 5 oz (140g) baby arugula (about 6 cups)
- 4 radishes, sliced
- ½ small red onion (sliced)

Directions

Step 1: lightly coat the grill rack with cooking oil and (refer to tips under more info to know how).

Step 2: cut each chicken breast horizontally; open and pound to a ½ inch thickness (chicken grills faster when split and pounded).

Step 3: with ½ tbsp coriander, ¼ tsp pepper and ½ tsp salt season the chicken breast and grill on a high heat until cooked, about 3 minutes on each side.

Step 4: in a large bowl combine the arugula, radishes and onion followed by the oil, ½ teaspoon salt, and ¼ teaspoon pepper, lemon juice and toss to combine.

Step 5: serve the chicken on a plate toping it with the arugula salad

Dinner

Grilled Pork Chops with Cilantro Salsa

Serves: 6 (1 pork chop + 1/3 cup salsa/serving)
Calories: 240

Ingredients
- 1 ½ cups cubed cantaloupe
- 1 cup chopped tomatoes
- ½ cup chopped green pepper
- 2 tbsp thawed limeade concentrate
- 2 tbsp minced cilantro (fresh)
- 2 tbsp chopped green onion
- ¼ tsp salt
- 6 bone-in pork loin chops (each about 7 ounces)

Directions
Step 1: combine the first 3 ingredients in a bowl.
Step 2: cover limeade, cilantro, onions, salt and leave to sit in the fridge until ready to serve.
Step 3: season the pork with peppers and set aside until ready.

Step 4: lightly coat the grill rack with cooking oil and (refer to tips under more info to know how).

Step 5: grill the pork over a medium heat, covered, for about 4- 5 minutes on each side or until the thermostat reads 145 *c (290 *F) from the chops then leave to cool.

Step 3: serve the chops on a plate with the salsa and enjoy.

Farfalle with Chicken and Pesto

Serves: 4
Calories: 539

Ingredients
- 8 oz (225g) farfalle
- 1/2 cup reserved pasta water
- 1/2 lb. fresh green beans, ends trimmed
- 2 cups prepackaged grilled chicken
- 1/2 cup reduced-fat pesto sauce

Directions

Step 1: cook pasta as instructed by package directions.

Step 2: Reserve half cup pasta water after draining.

Step 3: in the meantime, in a shallow pan immerse the green beans and over a medium heat steam for 15 minutes.

Step 4: combine pesto, pasta, green beans, pasta water and chicken (cut into bite-size pieces) into a large bowl and stir until well mixed. Serve and enjoy!

Chapter 7: Success with the 5:2 Diet

The purpose of this book is to provide you with the right information that will guide you through the 5:2 diet. I'm assuming that you have a weight loss goal or goals that you would like to achieve. The 5:2 diet can help you achieve those goals and provide you with even more benefits. Using the information provided in the book so far will definitely bring results but in order to maximize your success I've added a few tips that should be helpful on your journey to a slimmer, healthier you.

Tip #1 – Say Bye to Junk Food

What's one thing that people have problems with when on a diet? Well, I can tell you more than one but temptation is something that is common with many diets especially at the beginning of their diets. It's true that you're only really dieting for 2 days in a week but having your favorite chocolate around on those days can make the day seem so much longer with that temptation. Now, some persons are able to tell themselves I'll have it tomorrow and eliminate that temptation but if you're not one of those people I suggest you get rid of the junk food, and quick.

Tip #2 – Drink Plenty of Water

Staying hydrated on fast days is important and drinking more than the usual recommendation of 8 glasses should be practiced. Why? On fast days there is no doubt that you are going to fill hungry and taking in plenty of water can reduce hunger pangs you might experience. This trick is used in many other diets. Also sometimes, depending on your eating habits your brain will confuse hunger for thirst when all that you need to do is drink more water. Consuming more water on fast days will give the impression that you are filled and have you handle the fast days easier than normal.

Tip #3 – Be Busy on Fast Days

It's no secret that people tend to eat when they're bored or just laying around doing nothing so you should try to avoid that as much as possible on fast days. Being busy on fast days will act as a distractions and the day will go by a lot quicker. If there are days in the week where you are busier than others try scheduling them as your fast days to see how it goes with you. From what I've seen and experienced for myself a busy fast day is a fast day well handled.

Tip #4 – Learn to Count Calories

The main thing about this diet is that on fast days you limit your calorie intake to no more than 500 calories and to do that you must be mindful of what you put into your body. In the previous chapters you have really great recipes that can make this simple for you as well as other food suggestions that can guide you along. However if you're looking for ways of calculating calorie intake there are many options online, a couple of which are my calorie counter and calorie king.

Tip #5 – Plan Ahead

Before your fast day begins you should have at least an idea of what you're going to eat and when for the day. This makes it less confusing and clearer for you. I don't think you would want to be in the fridge wondering what should I prepare when you're already hungry, now do you? A well planned day will make the experience easier and less frustrating.

Chapter 8: Frequently Asked Questions

Q. On what days during the week should I schedule my fast days?

1. In the book we mentioned that fast days should be non-consecutive but the main reason for that is to be able to get use to the diet and not place too much on the body at the beginning. Whether it's consecutive or non-consecutive it doesn't matter but most prefer non-consecutive. E.g. Monday and Thursday.

Q. Can I exercise on a fast day?

1. Studies that have been done has shown that people who exercise on fast days tend to burn more fat than usual so you can if you are interested. However, intense workouts should not be attempted and if for some reason you feel uncomfortable during your exercising, stop immediately.

Q. Are there any side effects to fasting?

1. The side effects that you experience during fasting are expected such as feeling hungry and that's only when you first start. Persons have reported that they get headaches and are sometimes constipated but I believe that's due to a lack of water during fast days.

Q. What do I do after I've gotten to my weight loss goal?

1. The 5:2 diet isn't something you do once and go back to your old habits, for most it's a way of life and if you've reached your goal and feel comfortable - no problem. To maintain your weight all you have to do is reduce on your fasting days to only once a week. That way you keep your-self looking great and in shape.

Q. What should I do if I'm not losing weight?

1. If you're not losing weight change the pattern. Try using 4:3 rather than 5:2 and see how that works for you. In other cases people might be putting back what they lost in the 5 days of

non-fasting so watch what you eat on non-fast days also. Try switching the non-so-healthy foods with the healthy ones.

Conclusion

It is my sincere hope that you might have liked all the recipes which have been mentioned in the book and once again thank you for getting this book and experimenting with the recipes.

About The Author

Marion Fields is born with the vision to promote *Intermittent fasting* among the masses. The author has written several research papers on the topic. He has served as an instructor promoting various cultural arts in University of San Francisco. He is currently living with his spouse in Texas.

www.ingramcontent.com/pod-product-compliance
Lightning Source LLC
LaVergne TN
LVHW012001070526
838202LV00054B/4993